S0-AKF-070

Thighs
to Die For

Thighs *to* Die For

BY ANN PICCIRILLO
WITH RUTH HARRIS

ILLUSTRATIONS BY KIM FRALEY

WORKMAN PUBLISHING • NEW YORK

Copyright © 1997 by Ann Piccirillo and Ruth Harris
Illustrations copyright © 1997 by Kim Fraley.

All rights reserved. No portion of this book may be reproduced—mechanically, electronically
or by any other means, including photocopying—without written permission of the publisher.
Published simultaneously in canada by Thomas Allen & Son Limited.

The Focus Weight cuff packaged with *Thighs to Die For* was designed by the author specifically for this
book. It is based on her Focus Weight® product.
Focus Weight® is a registered trademark of MB Focus, Inc.

Library of Congress Cataloging-in-Publication Data

Piccirillo, Ann
Thighs to die for : book and custom exercise pouch / by Ann Piccirillo, with Ruth Harris.

P. cm.

ISBN 0-7611-0556-5
1. Reducing exercises. 2. Thighs. I. Harris, Ruth, 1936–
II. Title.
RA781.6.P53   1997

613.7'1–dc21   97-2162

                                                                CIP

Workman books are available at special discounts when purchased in bulk for premiums and sales
promotions as well as for fund-raising or educational use. Special editions can also be created to
specification. For details, contact the Special Sales Director at the address below.

Workman Publishing Company
708 Broadway
New York, NY 10003-9555

Book printed and package assembled in the United States of America
Focus weight cuff manufactured in Hong Kong.
First printing May 1997

10 9 8 7 6 5 4 3 2 1

For Nicholas and Zoë

ACKNOWLEDGMENTS

I would like to thank all my clients for their years of support and express my gratitude to the staff at Manhattan Body for its loyalty and dedication.

Thanks to the editors and staff of Workman Publishing for their input and to my lawyer, Karen Shatzkin, for her help.

A great big thank-you to Dodie Kazanjian for the two witty and inspirational articles in *Vogue* that introduced me to millions of readers.

Special thanks to Ruth Harris for taking my ideas and putting them into words—there wouldn't be a book without her.

—A.P.

Focus Weight® is a registered trademark of MB Focus, Inc.

CONTENTS

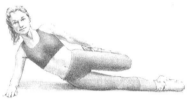

I Hate My Thighs! Can You Help Me? • Not All Bodies Are Created Equal • Not All Exercise Programs are Created Equal • What is a Healthy Body Image, and How Do I Get One? • Working Toward a Positive Body Image • The Thighs to Die For Program • Targeting Your Heart Rate

How the Focus Weight Theory Was Born • Goodbye Ankle Weights! Hello Focus Weights • Target and Tone • Know Your Thigh • Repeat and Resist • Preparing Your Focus Weight Cuff • Positioning Your Focus Weight Cuff • When to Exercise • Before You Start • Safety First • Listen to the Music • Warm-Up/Stretch, Cool-Down/Stretch • The Warm-Up • Stretching • Cooling Down

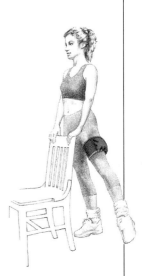

❏ FROM ME TO YOU: A PERSONAL NOTE

Perhaps you've read about the thigh-reduction program I developed that helped *Vogue* writer Dodie Kazanjian lose more than an inch off each thigh in less than a month. Perhaps you've heard about my exercise studio, Manhattan Body, located in New York City. Or perhaps you've picked up this book because you are unhappy about the shape and appearance of your own thighs and are looking for help.

Before I tell you how you can have the thighs of your dreams, I want to take this opportunity to introduce myself and tell you about the professional and personal experiences that led me to develop the Thighs to Die For Program.

I grew up on Long Island. I was a chubby and clumsy child when my parents enrolled me in ballet classes at the age of four. My early ballet training helped create the long, lean-lined body I enjoy today and also triggered an interest in dance, which I pursued throughout childhood and later in college at the Boston Conservatory of Music and Dance. Working at the barre, lined up in front of the all-seeing mirror and the pitiless eyes of my teachers, I learned the creed every dancer lives by: you can never be long enough, you can never be thin enough, and you can never be good enough.

Still young and impressionable, I took the constant criticism to heart and fell into the same trap most of my friends did: I began to compare myself to everyone else and incessantly berated myself for not being thin enough, long enough, and perfect enough. I became obsessed with my body and the flaws I perceived in it.

In a desperate attempt to 'measure up,' I resorted to diet pills, fasting, laxatives, and every fad diet that came along. Not surprisingly, I felt weak and found it difficult to get through a day of classes. I was tired; I couldn't concentrate; and, eventually, although I never became anorexic like many of my fellow dancers, I did stop menstruating.

Despite my desire to please my teachers and the mirror, I found the consequences of constant dieting tremendously debilitating, not only physically but psychologically. My relentless self-criticism and my efforts to maintain an unnaturally thin body through punitive starvation diets were undermining my confidence and distorting my sense of my own body image.

Much as I loved dance, I began to resent the demands for uniformity that the world of ballet imposed and started to question the rigid self-denial young dancers feel compelled to impose on themselves. I began to explore in greater depth the feelings and attitudes I was developing, and, over time, I gradually moved away from a career in dance. Instead, using my own experiences as a starting point, I studied exercise and nutrition and gravitated toward the healthier and more realistic approach that eventually became the cornerstone of my work.

I am now forty and have been a fitness instructor, owner of my own exercise studio, and, most recently, inventor of the Focus Weight cuff and the Thighs to Die For Program. In the past fifteen years I have worked with thousands of women of all shapes and sizes, teaching them how to stay trim without starvation and self-denial and how to exercise correctly and effectively.

The Thighs to Die For Program consists of three elements: aerobics to shed fat, body sculpting to shape the thigh, and food strategies to become, and stay, slim. In the pages that follow, I will focus on all three elements, but specifically the unique body sculpting plan and slimming food strategies I have developed over the years.

With this book comes an exercise aid for thighs called the Focus Weight cuff. This cuff is made up of elastic and Velcro panels that can be adjusted to fit on any thigh, and a pouch that can be filled with pennies to provide the exact amount of weight resistance you need. Everyone's thighs are different and everyone's goals are a little different, too, but with the Focus Weight cuff and the Thighs to Die For Program, you have everything you need to get slim, toned thighs.

As an integral part of my Thighs to Die For Program, the Focus Weight cuff will help you get the most out of each of the exercise routines. Placed on the precise thigh muscle to be toned, the weighted pouch acts as my hands guiding you into the correct positions as you exercise, showing you exactly which muscles to use. This simple device adds a whole new effectiveness to sculpting exercises. You will not be bored, you will not injure yourself, and you will not waste your time with exercises that don't help you achieve your goals.

Clients who have followed the Thighs to Die For Program have lost inches from their thighs safely, easily, and quickly without starving themselves or spending hours each day exercising. They are thrilled with their new look and feel liberated from the destructive self-criticism so many women fall prey to. What worked for them will work for you!

I have written this book in response to hundreds and hundreds of requests from my clients, from the readers of *Vogue*, and from women across the country who have heard about my success with others, and have designed this exercise cuff for *you*. It is my way of being there with you as you take the simple steps that will create the trim, toned thighs you have always wanted.

The words on these pages are my voice leading you along the way, carefully explaining the proper body positions, the best method of performing each part of the routine, and the goal of each exercise. I also explain in detail my simple but effective nutritional plan, which has worked for my many clients over the years. You will find the process interesting, enjoyable, and—best of all—effective!

I know you will love the results!

Ann Piccirillo

CHAPTER

1

GETTING STARTED

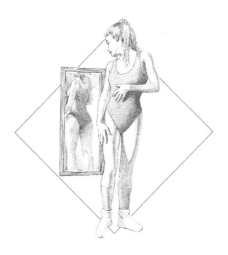

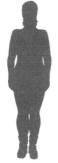

Ectomorph

Mesomorph

Endomorph

❏ I HATE MY THIGHS! CAN YOU HELP ME?

Yes! Absolutely, positively, *yes*. I can help you just as I have helped hundreds of women over the years. The Thighs to Die For Program is easy, safe, and inexpensive. There are no fads, no overnight "miracles," and no gimmicks. Best of all, it works.

Anyone, in any shape, will begin to feel the results in two weeks—or even sooner. Before we start, though, it is important to establish a positive attitude in order to approach your work in a commonsense, realistic way.

❏ NOT ALL BODIES ARE CREATED EQUAL

Ectomorph, mesomorph, and endomorph, the terms that classify the three basic body types, may be words that you have heard but do not exactly understand. Each of us is primarily one of them. *Ectomorphs*, or "string beans," tend to be lean and have long arms and legs. They have difficulty in acquiring muscular definition but little problem in losing body fat. *Mesomorphs* tend to be strong and naturally muscular. They have little difficulty in developing muscle definition and their weight tends to be within normal ranges. *Endomorphs*, sometimes referred to as "apples" or "pears," are round and soft in shape, carry their weight in the lower body, and have difficulty losing body fat.

These three body types are obviously different. Each stores fat differently, and each features a different level of muscle development. Your body type determines whether exercise or weight loss will be the more important factor in trimming and toning your thighs. The ectomorph needs to focus on exercise that will improve and enhance muscle definition; the mesomorph must be careful to avoid building excessive bulky muscle; the endomorph must concentrate on keeping her weight down while firming and contouring her muscles.

Aside from having one or another of the basic body types, women are faced with two additional physical realities that affect the size and shape of our thighs. Our bodies normally have a higher proportion—18–22%—of fat than men, whose normal range is from 12–17%. And women tend to gather weight on our lower bodies as a reserve for the calorie-intensive task of childbearing.

While we cannot change our heredity or the natural tendency of our particular body type any more than we can add inches to our height, we *can* modify the proportions we were born with. Simple nutritional modifications along with a well-thought-out program of exercise can do a great deal to close the gap between the body you see in the mirror and the body you want.

❏ NOT ALL EXERCISE PROGRAMS ARE CREATED EQUAL

Women have come to me over the years, unhappy and frustrated because they have exercised diligently without seeing the results they had hoped for. They feel that they have wasted time and money on

> Everyone, regardless of genetic make-up, can improve their appearance through the combined effects of good nutrition and a properly conceived and executed exercise program.

> Many people have experienced frustration and failure in their attempts to achieve a better body because they don't know how to attain the desired results.

trendy exercise equipment and expensive gym memberships that haven't helped—and they are right. To be effective, exercise must be undertaken with a specific and realistic body goal in mind. It must be designed to achieve the desired shape, and it must be performed correctly.

Workouts are of two basic types—they can be focused on developing strength, or endurance. A workout whose goal is to develop strength, emphasizes heavy weights and few repetitions. Done conscientiously, such a workout achieves exactly what it promises: you will build strength, but you will also develop big, bulky muscles. An endurance-oriented workout utilizes lighter weights and more repetitions and will create leaner, longer-looking muscles.

These results occur because two types of muscle fibers are in use when you work out—fast-twitch muscle fibers and slow-twitch muscle fibers. The strength or muscle-building workout utilizes more fast-twitch muscle fibers. By using heavy weights in strenuous repetitions, the muscle fibers are continually contracted and rebuilt, resulting in a bulking-up of the muscle.

The strength-oriented workout feels strenuous and difficult. Gyms often promote this approach on the no-pain-no-gain theory and because many clients feel they are not getting anything out of their workout unless they struggle through it. There is nothing wrong with a workout whose goal is to develop muscle size, but it is important to understand that it is not suited for the woman who wants to shape up and trim down.

An endurance-oriented program emphasizes more slow-twitch muscle fibers and consists of working with

When you exercise regularly, you will see improvement in the efficiency with which your heart and lungs function—which in turn increases your body's ability to burn calories. You will notice a loss of body weight, a loss of body fat, and an increase in muscle and lean weight.

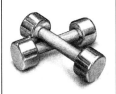

lighter weights and performing numerous repetitions of each exercise. Unlike the strength-oriented program, which enlarges muscles, the endurance-oriented program firms muscles, thus giving them a toned, lean look.

If you are accustomed to strength-oriented exercise, you may feel that the endurance workout isn't "hard" enough to give you the results you want. But it is the duration and the number of repetitions that create the long, lithe look you want. Just remember that a workout does not need to be grueling and you do not need to work yourself into a state of exhaustion to see results. The endurance-oriented workout is both challenging and effective, and it is the one that will best help you shape and streamline your thighs.

> The extent to which a woman can develop muscle tissue is determined by heredity, body build, and the intensity of her exercise program.

> Choose a program you can live with; if you don't, the changes you achieve will only be temporary.

❏ WHAT IS A HEALTHY BODY IMAGE, AND HOW DO I GET ONE?

Most of us, when we look in a mirror, can find something to criticize. According to the *American Journal of Psychiatry*, more than 70 percent of women are dissatisfied with their bodies. Too short, too tall, too thin, too fat—the list seems endless. It's not surprising, when you think of all the "glamorous" images women are bombarded with every day. Thousands of messages in the media reinforce unrealistic and even unhealthy standards of beauty. Despite common sense and scientific evidence to the contrary, women want to believe that, no matter what their age or genetic disposition, they can starve and mold themselves into the ultrathin

"I saw the difference in three days! And in less than a week I had lost half an inch off my waist and the same off my thighs. As I continued the Thighs to Die For Program, I looked and felt less bloated, and my thighs trimmed down and shaped up. I have struggled with weight all my life, and all I can say is that Ann Piccirillo's method is the only one that has ever worked for me."

—Susan A., 53

images relentlessly presented in the movies and by advertisers and fashion magazines.

Though this myth of the "perfect" body feeds the fitness industry of which I am a part, I must warn you that extreme thinness is not only an unattainable goal for most women but can also lead to unhealthy consequences, such as the eating disorders anorexia nervosa and bulimia.

The first step in any kind of body work is the development of a healthy body image. We already know that each body is different. What many of us haven't yet accepted is that each body can be beautiful—and by that I do not mean glamorous or model-perfect. I am referring to the authentic beauty that comes from confidence, energy, and feeling good about yourself. What you need to do—and what I will help you do—is change your image of yourself and then make *your* body the best it can be.

The challenge is to accept the body type you have and stop treating it as the enemy. Begin thinking of your body as your partner in this process, and be careful not to be overly critical of the way you look or unrealistic about how you think you should look. Start to treat yourself with compassion, and remember, as we proceed, that you will definitely have firm, toned, shapely thighs—thighs that are proportional to your frame and body type. Our goal is not some unrealistic fantasy of perfection but to sculpt *your* biological givens into the most attractive proportions possible.

You will work toward that goal day by day and step by step, but, before you start, I want to point out a trap that many women fall into. I have noticed over and over in my work that, even after there have been notice-able changes in their shape and muscle definition, many women still look in the mirror and see themselves as fat and unshapely. They see their progress as an acci-dent or a fluke and do not give themselves credit for their success.

To alter the way you see and feel about yourself, *you must be willing to acknowledge your improve-ments as they happen and to use your progress as motivation.* Make a conscious decision to free yourself from old, negative ways of viewing yourself. It's the only way that you will be able to take a realistic and encour-aging look at the changes you have made.

> While you keep your goal in mind, remember to enjoy the process.

❑ WORKING TOWARD A POSITIVE BODY IMAGE

The five practical suggestions that follow will help you replace the negative habits you may have fallen into with new, more positive attitudes toward yourself and your body.

1. Get rid of your scale. Your scale is not a friend; it's not even always truthful. Every woman knows that she can expect a slight weight gain around her period, and every woman knows that she is not defined by that small, normal variation, which is due to water retention or hormonal changes. Focusing on a number on the scale can be destructive psychologically and can lead to poor nutritional habits.

Don't use the numbers on the scale as a monitor of who you are or how well or poorly you are doing in life—or even to measure your progress as you follow this program.

Also, remember that a toned body can weigh more than an untoned body because muscle weighs more than fat. As you increase the ratio of muscle to fat, you may weigh a little more, but you are also increasing the rate at which your body uses calories. Studies have shown that as you build muscle, you increase the amount of metabolically active tissue, leading to a higher rate of caloric burn—another important reason to ignore your scale.

> Muscle tissue has a higher density than fat. As you shed fat and sculpt your muscles, the scales may not change drastically but your figure will improve dramatically.

Don't look at the scale. Look in the mirror!

2. Throw away your measuring tape. Half an inch on a measuring tape may not seem like very much, but it makes an enormous difference in the way your clothes fit. Obsessing over a number on a measuring tape is just as counterproductive as obsessing over a number on the scale, and you will accomplish little beyond making yourself miserable. Instead of relying on a measuring tape, use a tight-fitting skirt or pair of pants as a guide to judging your progress.

Each week, put on the same skirt or pair of pants and notice how it fits. When the button is more comfortable around the waist, when the buttocks no longer strain the seams, when your hips no longer pull at the sides of your skirt, when your pants begin to feel looser—that is proof positive that your body is changing shape and an inspiring way to keep yourself motivated from week to week.

3. Focus on your body—not your body parts. When you find yourself unhappy about your thighs, make a deliberate effort to interrupt the cycle of negative and self-critical thoughts. Focus instead on what you find attractive about yourself—your waist, your ankles, your hair, your eyes, your hands—and remind yourself that you are working to improve the part you don't find as attractive. I promise that very soon your thighs will be more in proportion to the rest of your body—and their significance will diminish in proportion in your mind.

4. Free yourself from media brainwashing. Models, television and film stars, and fashion magazines all give out the same message. Extreme thinness is the one and only way to be beautiful. It is important to remember that many models have naturally ectomorphic body types, and many also suffer from eating disorders. The actresses whose figures you admire adhere to rigid diets and spend thousands of dollars and many hours a day with personal trainers to achieve the ultrathin and sculpted look the camera demands. The time has come to stop comparing yourself to other women. Learn to be comfortable with your own body and the way it looks. Part of freeing yourself is to concentrate on replacing unachievable goals with attainable ones!

5. Take baby steps. You have had your thighs for years, and they have grown accustomed to your old habits. They will not change overnight, but, if you follow the Thighs to Die For Program, you can be sure they *will* change. Your body needs time to realize that it's been set on a new path, time to adjust to new habits of eating and exercising, and when it does—and it will—the results will follow.

9

In an era of instant gratification, body shaping is one of the last of the slow-but-sure accomplishments. Be patient, and remember that what seem to be small improvements will result in the big changes you want.

❏ THE THIGHS TO DIE FOR PROGRAM

Take advantage of the mind-body connection. Visualize the muscle you are working on and the shape you want to achieve as you exercise.

My thigh reshaping and recontouring program consists of three parts: aerobics to shed fat, body sculpting to shape, and food strategies to slim. These three elements work together to help you trim and tone your thighs quickly and effectively. To achieve your goals, you must combine *all three elements*.

Use Body Sculpting to Shape

Body sculpting is a term that describes the specific kind of exercise that creates shape. A toned muscle looks and feels strong and resilient whether you are actively working out or simply in a state of relaxation. Sculpting creates muscles that are shapely and firm to the touch, giving a longer, slimmer appearance.

To recontour the thighs, all four major muscle groups of the upper leg must be worked. It is on these four muscle groups that the program concentrates. Everyday activities such as walking and climbing stairs use the quadriceps (the long muscles that run down the front of the thigh) and hamstrings (the muscles on the back of the leg), but because of our national tendency toward inactivity, even these muscles are often untoned and out of shape. I know of no everyday movement that uses the muscles on the inner (adductors) and outer (abductors) thigh. These are the muscles whose shape we are most conscious of when we look straight ahead into a mirror, and, because they are almost completely unused, they are even more underdeveloped than the muscles on the front and back of the leg.

It is important to exercise all four muscle groups for both appearance and safety reasons. A leg with a highly developed outer thigh but weak inner thigh is unattractive because the outer portion of the thigh is firm and toned while the inner part is soft and flabby.

The muscles in your thigh act in pairs—inside/outside and front/back. The muscles in each pair oppose each other—when one contracts, the other lengthens. Exercising opposing muscle groups promotes muscle balance, thus preventing possible injury to the weaker muscle.

A well-thought-out program of body sculpting is essential to achieving long, lean muscles. These exercises must be carefully formulated and performed correctly in order to avoid building thick, bulky muscles that will make your legs look heavier. A routine consisting of less resistance, lighter weights, and more repetitions produces a slimmer and more contoured leg.

Use Aerobics to Shed

Aerobic exercise is oxygen-consuming activity involving the large muscle groups in continuous movement. During aerobic exercise, the breathing rate increases and the heart rate speeds up. The goal of aerobic exercise is to burn calories, thus reducing body weight and improving the appearance of your muscles by shedding the fat that obscures them. Moderate- to low-intensity,

Aerobics is an excellent method of improving your cardiovascular and respiratory systems, but a program of specific toning exercises is required to create a shapelier silhouette.

Reminder:

Depending on your body type, one aspect of the Thighs to Die For program will be more important to you than to someone else with a different body type. If you are an ectomorph, you may already be slim, so you will need to concentrate on sculpting exercises that create shape and definition. Mesomorphs will focus on keeping their weight within normal ranges while they use the exercise program to reshape their naturally larger muscles into leaner and longer proportions. If you are an endomorph, you will want to focus on the nutritional plan and the exercise program equally.

long-duration rhythmic exercise has been shown to be most effective in promoting body-fat loss. *Exercising for a longer time at 65% of your maximum heart rate is more effective in burning fat than shorter, more intense workouts.*

Outdoor jogging, step aerobics, stair climbing, walking or running on a treadmill, and riding a stationary bike are among the most popular aerobic workouts. However, because strenuous aerobic routines can also add bulk to the lower body, I advise clients to concentrate more on the duration of their workout and less on its difficulty. A lower-intensity workout allows you to increase the duration of your exercise.

If you use a treadmill, for example, walk at a brisk pace rather than jog or run. If you use an exercise bicycle, ride on flat terrain rather than up and down steep hills. On a stair climber, stick to shallower steps. Jogging, riding up and down hills, and steeper steps are strenuous and tend to develop large, strong muscles. Brisk walking, riding on a level pitch, and taking smaller steps create a longer, leaner look. For most healthy women, I recommend a 20- to 30-minute aerobic workout at target heart rate three times a week.

When doing the aerobic portion of this program, remember: concentrate on the *duration* of your workout, not its degree of difficulty.

Use Food Strategies to Slim

The last essential aspect of the Thighs to Die For program involves the kind and quantity of food you eat. The food pyramid published by the U.S. Department of Agriculture recommends 6 to 11 servings of bread,

TARGETING YOUR HEART RATE

To maximize the fat-burning results of your aerobic workout and get the full cardiovascular benefits of aerobic exercise, it is important to work at your target heart rate. Working within the target heart rate zone for a longer duration at a moderate intensity causes your body to get its fuel from fat. Working at a faster pace forces the body to rely on glycogen, the body's carbohydrate reserve, for energy.

Exceeding the target heart rate can be dangerous, while working below it will not achieve the fat-burning or cardiovascular results you want.

To determine your resting heart rate, place two fingers on your wrist directly below the base of your thumb and locate your pulse. Count how many times your heart beats in 10 seconds. Multiply this number by 6 and you know how many times your heart beats per minute. (The average resting heart rate for women is 78–84 beats per minute. A person in good aerobic condition generally has a lower resting heart rate.)

To find your maximum heart rate (the fastest your heart should beat) subtract your age from 226. To determine your target heart rate zone, take your maximum heart rate and multiply it by .55 and .75. Your heart rate during aerobic exercise should then fall within this range.

AGE:	55%	75%
20	113	154
25	111	151
30	108	147
35	105	143
40	102	140
45	100	136
50	97	132
55	94	128
60	91	125
65	89	121

To gain the benefits of aerobic exercise, it is important to keep the following three criteria in mind.

Frequency. The exercise should be performed from three to five times per week.

Duration. The exercise must last at least 20 minutes to achieve gains in aerobic endurance. More significant gains will occur with longer duration.

Intensity. Working at 55% to 75% of maximum heart rate range is considered ideal for healthy adults.

cereal, rice, or pasta per day. These tend to be filling foods and can cause you to feel bloated. I believe that the recommended quantity of these particular foods is excessive for the average woman, particularly those trying to slim down.

Carbohydrates are essential, and, while I am not advocating that you cut all carbohydrates out of your diet, I do propose that you limit the quantity and type you consume. Research has shown that the carbohydrates found in bread, cereal, pastas, and rice contribute to food cravings that result in the ingestion of excessive amounts of calories. If you are not an athlete or not involved in a very physically demanding lifestyle, these calories are not used by your body as fuel but are stored as fat. Which, thanks to biology, almost inevitably ends up where you least want it: on your hips, buttocks, and thighs!

CHAPTER

2

THE FOCUS WEIGHT THEORY

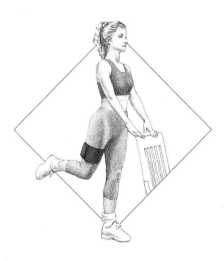

❏ HOW THE FOCUS WEIGHT THEORY WAS BORN

The Focus Weight theory evolved during my years of working with women who were unhappy with their thighs. I first began to develop the theory when I saw that although my clients were working hard trying to tone their thighs with traditional exercises and ankle weights, they weren't getting the results they wanted. Despite their efforts, my clients weren't trimming and toning the stubborn areas of their upper legs.

As I watched my classes, I began to see that clients struggled with three different kinds of problems. First, there were women who didn't know quite *where* the muscle they were supposed to be working was. Second, there were women who didn't know *how* to work the muscle. And third, there were women who wanted to work harder and, in the process of using a heavier ankle weight to intensify the workout, lost their focus on the thigh muscle to be toned and concentrated on the weight and the ankle instead.

I decided to figure out a way to solve all three problems at once. To help my clients exercise in the most effective way possible, I took a "hands-on" approach. I got rid of the ankle weights and placed my hands directly on the specific thigh muscle to be worked and, by pressing down slightly, created resistance during the "lifting" motion of the exercise. The feeling of my hand on the area to be toned instantly created a mind-body connection, locating the muscle for the client who wasn't quite sure where it was. That solved the first problem.

By pressing down, I encouraged the muscle to contract and to work in opposition to the resistance my hand created, thus helping the woman who wasn't sure how to work it. Problem two solved.

By removing the weight from the ankle and placing pressure on the thigh, I redirected the attention of the third type of client from her ankle to her thigh, the area she needed to work. Third problem solved.

This hands-on approach immediately helped my clients focus on the area they wanted to tone. The results were dramatic.

❏ GOOD-BYE ANKLE WEIGHTS! HELLO FOCUS WEIGHTS

Even though ankle weights have been used for years, I began to realize that they tended to prevent clients from working their thighs properly. Since ankle weights draw attention to the feet and ankles, they encourage lifting from the foot. Apart from being ineffective in trimming down the upper leg, lifting from the foot can cause the knee to rotate downward, thus throwing the leg out of alignment. When this happens, not only are the muscles of the upper leg unused, but, because the leg is out of position, the knee is unnaturally stressed and subject to injury. My clients were lifting from their feet and ankles—where they felt the weight—and not from the upper leg, the area they wanted to tone and shape. They had been wasting

"My skirts are looser and my thighs are definitely thinner! I've been very conscientious about the exercises and really enjoy doing them. I feel healthier, look better, and, best of all, I've lost inches from my thighs!"
—Janine S., 50

Fat and muscle are two different biological substances. Fat cannot be changed into muscle and muscle cannot be changed into fat.

their repetitions, but with my "hands on" approach, they *automatically* began to exercise correctly.

Although my hands-on approach was effective, it had its limitations because I could only work with one client at a time. I needed to find a way to give myself more than two hands! After several months of thinking and several more of experimenting, I created the Focus Weight as a way of replacing my hands. Rather than placing weight around the ankle where it distracted attention from the thigh, the Focus Weight is placed directly on the thigh and automatically positions resistance over the muscles to be toned.

In addition, the Focus Weight provides the correct amount of resistance in the right place, thus permitting the completion of many repetitions over a longer period of time.

The Focus Weight not only solved my problems, it also allowed me to put my endurance workout—less difficulty, longer duration—into practical application. Once I substituted the Focus Weight for ankle weights in my classes, my clients quickly began to see the changes they wanted.

❏ TARGET AND TONE

For years you have probably heard that it is impossible to reduce and/or change the shape of a specific body area. On the contrary, my experience has shown that it is perfectly possible to target and tone specific areas of the body. Using the Focus Weight and the Thighs to Die For Program, I have had gratifying success in helping all kinds of women dramatically improve the shape and appearance of their thighs.

I have worked with clients who have come to me with large, overdeveloped muscles and have helped them achieve a leaner and longer appearance. I have created and contoured shape in the legs of slender women who have never exercised before. I have reduced and reshaped the hips, thighs, and buttocks of women who tend to be naturally bottom-heavy. Even women who have exercised for years without seeing results have successfully recontoured and reproportioned their thighs. The light weight, the targeted exercises, and the multiple repetitions, together with aerobic exercise, will slim, tone, and shape the leg.

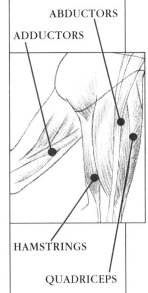

ABDUCTORS

ADDUCTORS

HAMSTRINGS

QUADRICEPS

❏ KNOW YOUR THIGH

Take a look at the diagram on this page and get to know your thigh. There are four major muscle groups in each thigh. They consist of the quadriceps in front, the hamstring in back, the abductors on the outer thigh, and the adductors on the inner thigh. These are some of the largest muscles in your body.

All muscles in your body work in pairs—while one muscle lengthens, its partner contracts. As you lift your leg in front, the quadriceps on the front of your thigh contract and the hamstring at the back of your thigh lengthens. When you lift your leg to the side, you contract your abductors and lengthen your adductors. It's important to work both partners in each muscle pair to sculpt the four major thigh areas equally.

❏ REPEAT AND RESIST

Don't let your body beat you. When you feel you can't go on, try to do one more repetition.

Focused repetitions and focused resistance are the keys to reshaping the upper leg. It is important not to waste your repetitions and it is essential that your thigh do all the work on every repetition for you to get the most out of each exercise. The Focus Weight guarantees the effectiveness of each repetition by concentrating weight on the specific muscle you want to tone and trim, allowing you to concentrate on that muscle each time you lift your leg. Resistance (the light downward pressure exerted by the Focus Weight) encourages the specific thigh muscle that the weight is directly over to contract. This combination of focused repetitions and focused resistance maximizes the effects of your workout, thus creating tone and shape.

❏ PREPARING YOUR FOCUS WEIGHT CUFF

I designed the Focus Weight cuff specifically for this book. It consists of an adjustable cuff that wraps around your thigh and a pouch that you fill with pennies to create a weight—the number of pennies that you use depends on your fitness level.

Start out with a 2-pound weight. Fill a plastic baggie with pennies ($3.50 worth) and secure the opening. Then place the bag into the pouch of the Focus Weight cuff. You can put anything that weighs about 2 pounds into the pouch.

❏ POSITIONING YOUR FOCUS WEIGHT CUFF

Place the weight at the midway point between your knee and your hip over the particular muscle group (outer thigh, inner thigh, front or back of thigh) you want to work, as shown in the drawings. The midpoint of the muscle is called the "belly" of the muscle. It is here that you want to focus your attention and effort as you exercise. By placing the Focus Weight cuff at the midpoint between the hip and the knee, you avoid the possibility of injury to either joint. In addition, the placement of the weight directly on the thigh encourages correct alignment and automatically helps you focus on the exact muscles you want to tone and the areas you want to reshape.

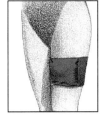

Once you have placed the weighted pouch over the thigh muscle to be worked, you'll secure the cuff with Velcro so it won't slip while you exercise. When the exercise cuff is in position, you will see and feel the weight on the area you want to sculpt. Use these two senses—sight and touch—to help you perform the exercises correctly.

If you are a beginner and have never exercised, or have never exercised using weights, you may find 2 pounds a bit heavy. In that case, remove half the filling ($1.75) from the bag, reseal, and put the bag back into the pouch. The pouch should weigh about 1 pound. Your lifts should feel comfortable—that is, you should be able to lift your leg with ease as you begin your workout. If there is still too much weight, remove more pennies until you find a satisfactory level. Your

"Within three weeks of starting the "Thighs to Die For" program my thighs had come down a whole inch. I went from size 14 pants to a size 10. For me, the "Thighs to Die For" program was the answer to a lifelong problem."

—Louise H., 58

goal is to be able to start your workout with the amount of resistance that is appropriate for you. Then you add more weight as your leg gets stronger.

If you are an experienced exerciser, accustomed to working with heavier weights, you may find that the 2-pound pouch feels light at first. Remember that many repetitions will cause a lighter weight to feel heavier. However, if you would like to try using a 3-pound weight, add another $1.75 to the pouch.

❏ WHEN TO EXERCISE

Choose a time of day to do your exercises and do your best to stick with your schedule. A regular routine will help you integrate exercise into your everyday life. Exercising in the morning will give you energy to start the day. Working out at midday will recharge your batteries. Doing your routine in the evening will release the tensions of the day and give you an opportunity to move if you have spent hours sitting.

❏ BEFORE YOU START

Before you exercise, you'll need to put on something comfortable and nonrestrictive, such as sweats, a T-shirt and shorts, or tights and a leotard. You might want to layer your clothes so that you can remove items easily if you get too hot.

It's important to wear the right shoes when you work out—especially in the aerobic portion of your routine. A cross-training sneaker is appropriate for both

SAFETY FIRST

Because of the positioning of the Focus Weight cuff, most people can do the exercises safely without stressing or injuring the knee. The following tips will also help you exercise effectively and safely.

1. Before beginning this or any other fitness program, consult your physician.

2. If you are a beginner and experience soreness, perform the exercises every other day until the muscles are stronger and the soreness disappears. Your goal is to build up the strength to do the exercises every day. If you feel stiff, a warm bath will help relax your muscles.

3. Be sure to follow the instructions for the warm-ups and cool-downs. They are an essential part of the Thighs to Die For Program and will help maintain your flexibility.

your aerobic workout and the toning program. This kind of shoe gives you support and prevents you from slipping.

The exercises are done sitting, lying on the floor, or standing, using a chair as a prop. For the floor exercises, place a towel or a mat on the floor to provide a bit of padding. For the exercises requiring a chair, use one with a back that is at a comfortable height to give you support and help you with balance. If convenient, exercise in front of a mirror so that you can check your posture and alignment.

You may want to use a towel or a mat for padding when you do the floor exercises.

23

❏ LISTEN TO THE MUSIC

Music is inspiring, and it can also make all aspects of your workout more fun. The tempo for each part of your workout will vary, but always be sure to choose pieces with a steady beat.

Music for the warm-up/stretch and cool-down/stretch should be slower and more relaxing than the music for the aerobic and toning portions of your workout. Music for the aerobic portion should be about 140 to 160 beats per minute. The best tempo for the body sculpting part of your program is about 120 beats per minute, or 2 beats per second.

Let the music move you. Strong rhythm will help you power your leg lifts.

❏ WARM-UP/STRETCH, COOL-DOWN/STRETCH

Always warm up and stretch before you begin to exercise, and, when you are finished, take a few moments to cool down and stretch. Warm-ups, cool-downs, and stretching are important ways to ease your body into and out of exercise safely.

The warm-up is the gradual transition from a resting to a working state; it prepares your body for the challenge of exercise by increasing your heart rate and speeding up blood flow to muscles and tendons, raising their temperature and increasing their flexibility. Loose, warm muscles are less likely to be strained, pulled, or injured.

❏ THE WARM-UP

The following warm-up exercises increase your heart rate and prepare your muscles for work. This routine should last from 9 to 15 minutes.

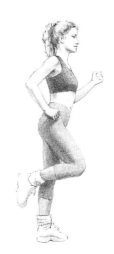

1. Jog in place for 3 to 5 minutes, moving your arms in a pumping motion.

2. March in place for 3 to 5 minutes, raising your knees to hip level and moving your arms in large, sweeping motions.

3. From a standing position, lean on one leg and reach up with the opposite hand. Alternate from side to side for 3 to 5 minutes.

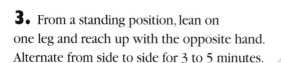

❏ STRETCHING

Stretching elongates muscles and encourages flexibility. At the beginning of a workout, stretching helps loosen muscles and prevent injury. At the end of your routine, stretching reduces muscle tension and stiffness. In addition, it eases the muscles you have been tightening and contracting during the workout. Concluding your workout with a stretch phase also lets your heart rate descend gradually and naturally.

The following exercises stretch the four specific areas of the thigh. Use them in both the warm-up and cool-down portions of your workout. Hold each stretch for at least 30 seconds. Breathe slowly and deeply as you stretch gently. Don't bounce or force any of the stretches—it's possible to pull or even tear muscles by stretching too far too fast.

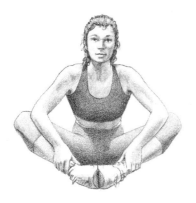

INNER THIGH STRETCH
(ADDUCTORS)

Sitting on the floor, place the soles of your feet together in front of you and place your hands on your ankles. Keeping your back straight, lean forward with your upper body and press your knees down and out to the side. Hold this position for 30 seconds.

BACK OF THIGH
STRETCH (HAMSTRINGS)
Sitting on the floor, extend both legs out straight in front of you. Lean forward with your upper body, reaching your hands out toward your ankles. Hold this position for 30 seconds.

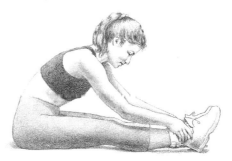

OUTER THIGH AND SADDLEBAG STRETCH

(ABDUCTORS/GLUTEUS MEDIUS)

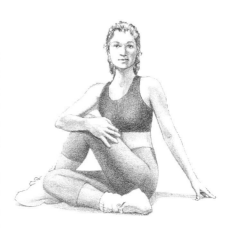

Sitting on the floor, bend your left leg in front of you. Cross your right leg over your left thigh, placing you right foot on the floor. Place your right hand on the floor by your side and wrap your left hand around the top of your right knee. Sitting up straight and twisting your torso to the right, pull your right knee into your chest as close as possible. Hold this position for 30 seconds. Repeat with the other leg.

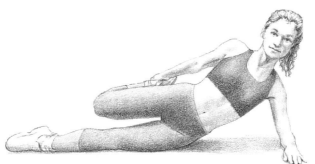

FRONT OF THIGH STRETCH

(QUADRICEPS)

Lie on your left hip and elbow and extend your legs out to the side. Keeping your left leg straight, bend your right knee and grasp the right foot, pulling it toward your buttocks. Keep your legs close together. Gently pull back on your right leg while pressing your hips forward. Hold this position for 30 seconds. Repeat with the other leg.

❏ COOLING DOWN

After every workout it is important to cool down. This reverses the process of the warm-up and helps speed muscle recovery by removing lactic acid, a metabolic by-product of exercise, that can cause pain or soreness if allowed to accumulate in the muscles and bloodstream.

As a cool down routine after each workout, per-form the warm-up and stretching exercises (pages 25–27) to bring your heart rate back to resting. Hold each stretch for 30 seconds on each leg.

Always stretch before and after you workout.

CHAPTER
3

THE
EXERCISES

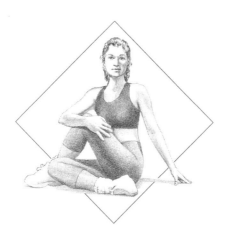

"I lost a half an inch from my thighs in less than two weeks! Ann Piccirillo's Thighs To Die For Program theory gave me the toned, leaner shape I've been wanting. It was easy and fit into my busy lifestyle without the slightest problem."

—Carol, 54

❏ VARIETY: THE SPICE OF LIFE

Variety in your exercise routine is important for a number of reasons, both mental and physical. First of all, it prevents boredom and helps you stay motivated. It also provides consistent physical challenge, helping you develop muscle strength. After a muscle becomes used to a particular exercise, challenge yourself and vary your workout with alternating routines.

The three workouts in this chapter call for different body positions and provide escalating degrees of challenge. Exercises performed lying on the floor are the easiest because the upper body is supported. Exercises done on all fours are more difficult because the upper body is engaged. Standing exercises are the most difficult because they require balance plus an erect posture, thus involving both upper-and lower-body strength.

❏ HOW OFTEN AND HOW LONG TO EXERCISE

The Thighs to Die For body sculpting program should take approximately 20 minutes and should be done daily to achieve optimum results. Start with the first workout variation and do *all five* of the exercises described. The purpose for everyone—beginner, intermediate, and advanced exercisers—is to challenge

FINDING YOUR FITNESS LEVEL

To find your fitness level, begin with the quadriceps exercise on page 36 and do as many repetitions as you can until you feel the muscle begin to fatigue. Then consult the following chart to find out whether you are at a beginning, intermediate, or advanced level.

Later, when the exercise becomes comfortable and you no longer feel challenged, add more repetitions to your routine. I suggest adding repetitions in sets of 8 to a maximum of 56. When you have mastered 56 repetitions, proceed to the variation at the next level of difficulty. When you can do all three variations easily, you are free to choose whichever variation you prefer or to do a different variation every day.

NUMBER OF REPETITIONS	FITNESS LEVEL
8–16	Beginner
16–32	Intermediate
32–56	Advanced

the muscles and increase strength with more and more repetitions.

Once you have determined your fitness level, you will have a good idea where to begin. As your legs get stronger, you will increase the repetitions.

Posture is one of the most underappreciated aspects of improved appearance. Proper alignment—torso aligned directly over hips, rib cage lifted, shoulders relaxed and down, abdominals contracted, pelvis slightly tucked—automatically makes one appear taller and slimmer, enhances the bustline, expands the chest, flattens the stomach, and lifts the buttocks.

❏ EXERCISE BASICS: POSTURE, TEMPO, AND BREATH

There are three things to remember when you are doing the exercises in the Thighs to Die For program—posture, tempo, and breath. Proper body alignment, exercise rhythm, and breathing all contribute to the efficiency of each exercise.

Posture—Body Alignment Maintaining good posture is crucial for two reasons: to prevent injury and to get the most benefit out of your repetitions. As you work, concentrate on keeping your shoulders down, your back straight, and your abdominals in. Keep your torso still as you perform the exercises in order to create the most resistance for each repetition.

Tempo—Lift, Lower, Pulse, and Squeeze
Exercise to an even, rhythmic tempo—I recommend a 2-count lift and a 2-count lower—so that the muscles have time to contract and release during each repetition. Each 2-count movement should take about 2 seconds. The term "pulse" indicates a small, more rapid 1-count-up and 1-count-down movement. Each pulse lasts for about a second. Squeeze and hold whichever muscle you are working for 4 counts during the pause in each exercise. Your goal is to complete each movement smoothly and fully, giving the muscle adequate time to contract and then to lengthen to its full extent. Moving in quick, staccato bursts lessens the effectiveness of exercise and can result in pulled or torn muscle tissue.

Breath—Remember to Breathe! Be sure to breathe throughout your exercise routines! An even flow of oxygen keeps your body relaxed and prevents you from becoming tense. You should breathe regularly and consistently. The level of activity will control the rate and depth of your breathing, so you will naturally breathe faster during the aerobic portions of your workout than during the toning periods.

❏ ACCENT UP/ACCENT DOWN

In a movement that is accented on the upward phase, the *concentric,* or positive, contraction is emphasized. This type of contraction shortens the muscles and occurs when you lift the weight. The *eccentric,* or negative, contraction lengthens the muscle as you lower the weight. This type of contraction occurs on the downward phase of a movement. Accenting both types of contractions during exercise is very effective in building strength and helps create an attractive shape.

❏ REPETITIONS AND INTERVALS

Sets of 8 repetitions are suggested because exercise is more enjoyable when done to music and most music is written in multiples of 8 beats. An interval with a resting *pause* between sets helps to reduce muscle fatigue in a workout that consists of many repetitions of the same muscle groups. In addition, when a muscle is weak, the pause gives the muscle a chance to recover before working again and helps prevent injury.

WORKOUT #1: FLOOR EXERCISES

This is the easiest of the three workouts because the floor exercises are done in a sitting, prone, or side-lying position. You will need an exercise mat or a towel. Do all the exercises with your right leg first. Then switch legs and perform all the exercises with your left leg.

Before you begin, make sure to do a proper warm-up and stretch as described on pages 25-27, and have completed the aerobic portion of your workout (if it's an aerobic workout day).

SCHEDULE AND ROUTINE

Warm-up/stretch	3–5 minutes daily
Aerobic activity	20–30 minutes, 3 times a week
Body sculpt	20 minutes daily
Repetitions	8–56 for each exercise
Cool-down/stretch	3–5 minutes daily

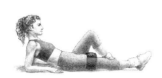 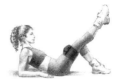

FRONT OF THIGH (Quadriceps)

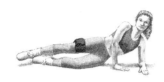 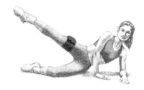

OUTER THIGH (Abductors)

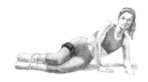 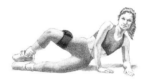

SADDLEBAG (Gluteus Medius)

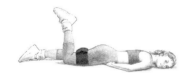 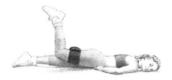

BACK OF THIGH (Hamstrings)

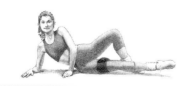 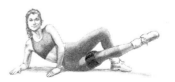

INNER THIGH (Adductors)

FRONT OF THIGH
QUADRICEPS

Step One
WEIGHT PLACEMENT

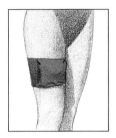

Place the weighted pouch of the Focus Weight cuff on the front of your right thigh midway between the knee and hip. Secure it snugly so that it won't slip while you exercise.

ALIGNMENT: In the sitting position, keep your upper torso erect, your rib cage lifted, and your shoulders back. For this exercise, keep the nonworking leg bent and the nonworking foot flat on the floor. Remember to contract the abdominals!

Step Two
THE MOVEMENT

A. Sitting on the floor, lean back on your elbows. Bend your left knee, placing the foot on the ground, and extend your right leg.

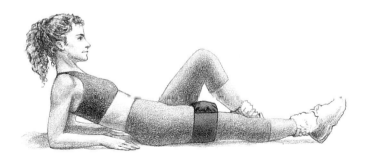

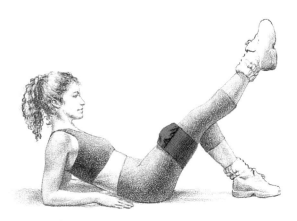

B. Without bending your right knee, lift your right leg until it is level with your left knee. Do not alter your upper body position. Pause.

Then lower your right leg to the floor.

TIP: Use slow, controlled movements to perform the leg lifts. Lift your working leg to knee height but no higher—this will help isolate the quads and lessen strain on your hip flexors.

Step Three
THE REPETITIONS

- Repeat the full range of motion 8 times, accenting the *up* movement of your leg.

- Lift your right leg to your left knee. Maintaining this height and with a small range of motion, *pulse* your leg up and down 8 times. The pulsing movement is small, ranging from your left knee down about 3 inches.

- As you become stronger, increase the pulses to a maximum of 54.

- Lower and lift your leg 8 times in the full range of motion, accenting the *down* movement.

- *Hold* your leg up for 4 counts.

OUTER THIGH
ABDUCTORS

Step One:
FOCUS WEIGHT PLACEMENT

Place the weighted pouch of the Focus Weight cuff on the outside of your right thigh midway between the knee and the hip. Secure it snugly so that it won't slip while you exercise.

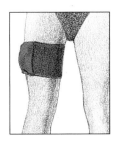

ALIGNMENT: Raise your body up on one elbow with your supporting arm positioned directly under your shoulder. Your rib cage should be lifted so that the torso does not collapse and your hips should be aligned one on top of the other perpendicular to the floor; they should not lean to the front or the back. The bottom leg is for support only, and the top leg should be extended in line from the hip.

Step Two
THE MOVEMENT

A. Lie on your left hip and elbow with your left leg bent. Fully extend your right leg at hip level.

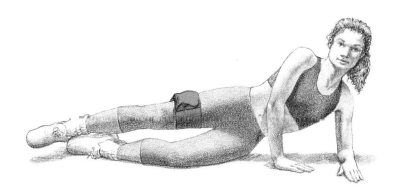

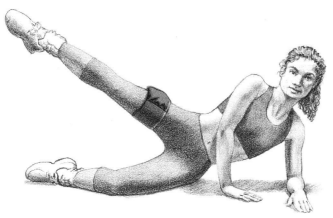

B. Lift your right leg up as high as you can, keeping your hips in a straight line, perpendicular to the floor. Pause.

Then lower your leg to within a few inches from the floor. Do not let your foot rest on the floor in the down position.

Step Three:

THE REPETITIONS

- Repeat the full range of motion 8 times, accenting the *up* movement of your leg.

- Lift your right leg to hip level. Maintaining this height and with a small range of motion, *pulse* your leg up and down 8 times.

- As you become stronger, increase the pulses to a maximum of 54.

- Lower and lift your leg 8 times in the full range of motion, accenting the *down* movement.

- *Hold* your leg up for 4 counts.

> **TIP:** Lift your leg as high as possible without altering alignment. Your knee should not rotate to the front or back but face directly forward to avoid involving your quads or hip rotators.

SADDLEBAG
GLUTEUS MEDIUS

Step One:
FOCUS WEIGHT PLACEMENT

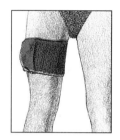

Place the weighted pouch of the Focus Weight cuff on the outside of your right thigh midway between the knee and the hip. Secure it snugly so that it won't slip while you exercise.

ALIGNMENT: Your supporting elbow should be placed on the floor directly under your shoulder. Be sure not to slouch! Your legs should be aligned so that the knees can rest directly on top of each other and the feet can stay touching.

Step Two:
THE MOVEMENT

A. Lie on your left hip and elbow with both legs bent to a 45-degree angle.

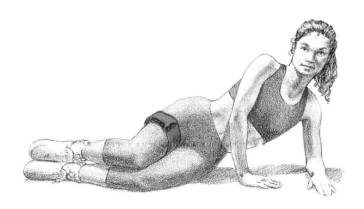

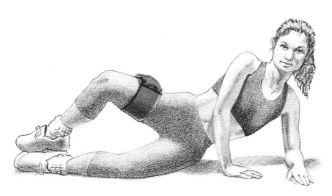

B. With your feet touching, open your right leg as wide as you can without sitting back into your hips. Pause.

Then lower your leg to the starting position.

Step Three:

REPETITIONS

• Repeat the full range of motion 8 times, accenting the *up* movement of your leg.

• Open your right leg as wide as you can. Maintaining this height and with a small range of motion, *pulse* your leg up and down 8 times.

• As you become stronger, increase the pulses to a maximum of 54.

• Lower and lift your leg 8 times in a full range of motion, accenting the *down* movement.

• *Hold* your leg up for 4 counts.

> **TIP:** In order to create the necessary amount of resistance between your leg and your hip, don't roll back onto the buttocks when opening your top leg.

41

BACK OF THIGH
HAMSTRINGS

Step One:
FOCUS WEIGHT PLACEMENT

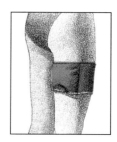

Place the weighted pouch of the Focus Weight cuff on the back of your right thigh midway between the knee and the hip. Secure it snugly so that it won't slip while you exercise.

ALIGNMENT: In the prone position, your chest should remain in contact with the floor and your hips should remain in contact with your hands. Keep your head in a comfortable position, laterally rotated to face sideways. Your working leg should remain in a 90° angle throughout the exercise.

Step Two:
THE MOVEMENT

A. Lie on your stomach. Place your hands under your hipbones. Bend your right leg at a 90° angle.

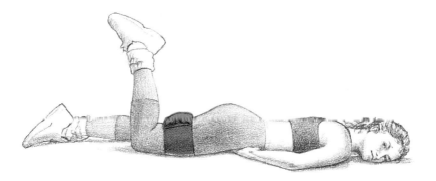

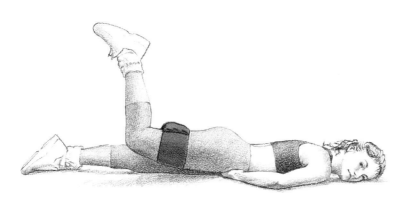

B. Lift your right leg a few inches off the floor, keeping your hips on your hands.

Pause. Then lower your right leg to the floor.

> **TIP:** The range of motion is limited by the prone position. In order to avoid hyper-extending your back, do not raise your leg above your buttocks.

Step Three
REPETITIONS

• Repeat the full range of motion 8 times, accenting the *up* movement of your leg.

• Lift your right leg a few inches from the floor. Maintaining this height and with a small range of motion, *pulse* your leg up and down 8 times.

• As you become stronger, increase the pulses to a maximum of 54.

• Lower and lift your leg 8 times in the full range of motion, accenting the *down* movement.

• *Hold* your leg up for 4 counts.

INNER THIGH
ADDUCTORS

Step One:
WEIGHT PLACEMENT

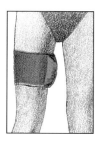

Place the weighted pouch of the Focus Weight cuff on the inside of your right thigh midway between the knee and the hip. Secure it snugly so that it won't slip while you exercise.

ALIGNMENT: When working on your side with your torso raised, do not collapse into the rib cage, especially as the lower leg is lifted. The top leg is bent in a supportive position while the lower leg should be extended in line with the hip.

Step Two:
MOVEMENT

A. Lie on your right hip and elbow. Bend your left knee, placing the foot on the floor, and extend and rotate your right leg out.

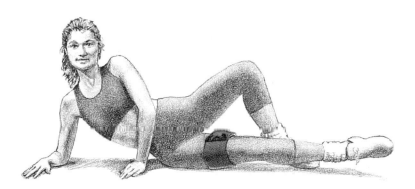

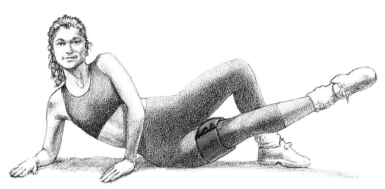

B. Lift your right leg level with your left calf without rolling back on your hip. Pause.

Then lower your right leg to within a few inches from the floor. Do not let your foot rest in the down position.

Step Three:
REPETITIONS

- Repeat the full range of motion 8 times, accenting the *up* movement of your leg.

- Lift your right leg to your left calf. Maintaining this height and with a small range of motion, *pulse* your leg up and down 8 times.

- As you become stronger, increase the pulses to a maximum of 54.

- Lower and lift your leg 8 times in the full range of motion, accenting the *down* movement.

- *Hold* your leg up for 4 counts.

> **TIP:** Be sure not to turn the toes of your working leg upward in order to avoid involving the quads. Do not allow your toes to turn downward to avoid involving your hamstrings.

Now that you have finished your right-leg workout, move the weight to your left leg and repeat the exercises. To cool down when you have completed the exercises with both legs, perform the stretching exercises described on pages 26–27.

WORKOUT #2: ALL-FOURS EXERCISES

The following exercises are done in the all-fours position except the one for the quadriceps (front of thigh), which is done in a sitting position. In the all-fours position, keep your abdominals contracted to prevent your lower back from hyperextending. In the sitting position, keep your back straight and your shoulders down.

For this workout, you will need an exercise mat or a towel.

Do all the exercises with your right leg first. Then switch legs and perform all the exercises with your left leg.

Before you begin, make sure you have had a proper warm-up/stretch and have completed the aerobic portion of your workout.

SCHEDULE AND ROUTINE

Warm-up/stretch	3–5 minutes
Aerobic activity	20–30 minutes, 3 times a week
Body sculpt	20 minutes daily
Repetitions	8–56 for each exercise
Cool-down/stretch	5–8 minutes

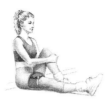 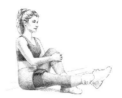

FRONT OF THIGH (Quadriceps)

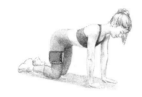 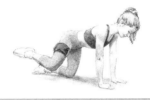

OUTER THIGH (Abductors)

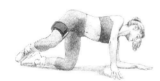 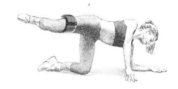

SADDLEBAG (Gluteus Medius)

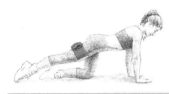 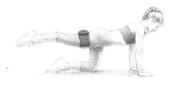

BACK OF THIGH (Hamstrings)

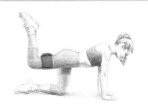 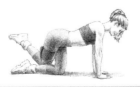

INNER THIGH (Adductors)

47

FRONT OF THIGH
QUADRICEPS

Step One:
WEIGHT PLACEMENT

Place the weighted pouch of the Focus Weight cuff on the front part of your right thigh midway between the knee and the hip. Secure it snugly so that it won't slip while you exercise.

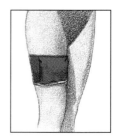

ALIGNMENT: Use the wall as your guide to correct body alignment. Contract your abdominals and gently press your lower back and shoulders against the wall. Maintain this position as you move the working leg up and down. Use the bent leg as support.

Step Two:
MOVEMENT

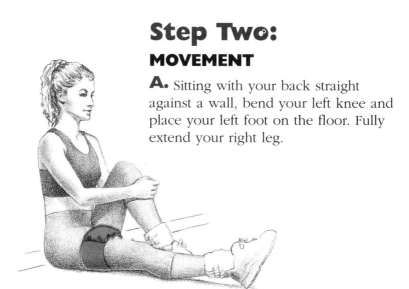

A. Sitting with your back straight against a wall, bend your left knee and place your left foot on the floor. Fully extend your right leg.

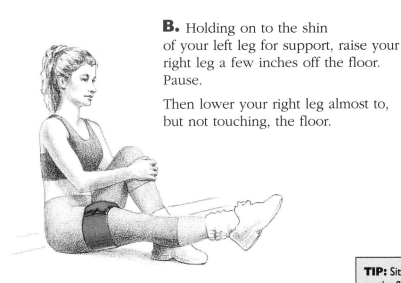

B. Holding on to the shin of your left leg for support, raise your right leg a few inches off the floor. Pause.

Then lower your right leg almost to, but not touching, the floor.

TIP: Sitting upright on the floor and maintaining an erect position is difficult, so expect even the full range of motion to be limited. Work in small movements to decrease the strain on your hip flexor.

Step Three:

REPETITIONS

• Repeat the full range of motion 8 times, accenting the *up* movement of your leg.

• Lift your right leg a few inches from the floor. Maintaining this height and with a small range of motion, *pulse* your leg up and down 8 times.

• As you become stronger, increase the pulses to a maximum of 54.

• Lower and lift your leg 8 times in the full range of motion, accenting the *down* movement.

• *Hold* your leg up for 4 counts.

OUTER THIGH
ABDUCTORS

Step One:
WEIGHT PLACEMENT

Place the weighted pouch of the Focus Weight cuff on the outside of your right thigh midway between the knee and the hip. Secure it snugly so that it won't slip while you exercise.

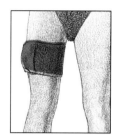

ALIGNMENT: On all fours, the knees should be separated and aligned under the hips. Hands should be directly under the shoulders. The hands and fingers should face forward. Hold the head in a natural extension of the spine; do not let it hang down. The abdominals should be contracted at all times in order to prevent the lower back from swaying.

Step Two:
THE MOVEMENT

A. Kneel in an all-fours position, placing your hands directly under your shoulders.

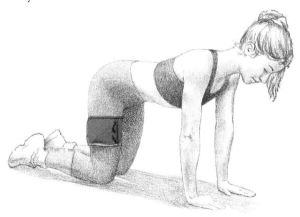

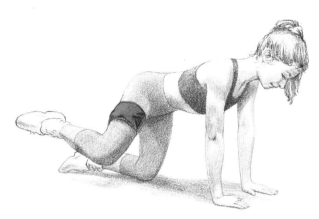

B. Keeping your hips and shoulders parallel to the floor, open your right leg directly out to the side as high as you can without lifting your right hip. Your hips should always be parallel to the floor and your working leg should always be bent at a 90° angle. Pause.

Then return your right leg to the starting position.

Step Three:
REPETITIONS

- Repeat the full range of motion 8 times, accenting the *outward* movement of your leg.

- Open your right leg out to hip level. Maintaining this height and with a small range of motion, *pulse* your leg out and in 8 times.

- As you become stronger, increase the pulses to a maximum of 54.

- Close and open your leg 8 times in the full range of motion, accenting the *inward* movement.

- On the last repetition, *hold* your leg open to the side for 4 counts.

TIP: When lifting your working leg, be sure to raise it directly to the side, leaving the knee facing forward. Keep your hips square and do not lean over onto your supporting leg. Hold your torso motionless in order to isolate your working leg.

SADDLEBAG
GLUTEUS MEDIUS

Step One:
FOCUS WEIGHT PLACEMENT

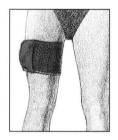

Place the weighted pouch of the Focus Weight cuff on the outside of your right thigh midway between the knee and the hip. Secure it snugly so that it won't slip while you exercise.

ALIGNMENT: In this exercise the all-fours position is slightly modified by lowering onto one elbow. This position allows for a greater range of motion. Do not slouch onto the supporting side, and keep the abdominals contracted.

Step Two:
MOVEMENT

A. Kneel in an all-fours position, placing your hands directly under your shoulders. Bend your left arm and place your left elbow on the floor. Keeping your feet together, open your right leg to a 45° angle.

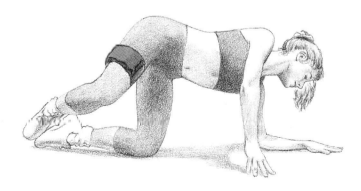

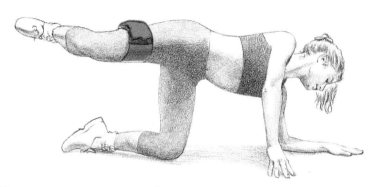

B. Lift your right leg up to hip level. Pause.

Then return your right foot to touch your left foot, leaving your leg open at a 45° angle.

Step Three:
REPETITIONS

> **TIP:** Do not lift your leg higher than the hip or your buttocks will do the work rather than your outer thigh.

- Repeat the full range of motion 8 times, accenting the *up* movement of your leg.

- Maintaining the 45° angle, lift your right leg to hip level. At this height and with a small range of motion, *pulse* your leg up and down 8 times.

- As you become stronger, increase the pulses to a maximum of 54.

- Leaving your right leg open at a 45° angle, return the right foot to touch the left foot. Pause. Then lift your right leg up to hip level. Repeat the full range of motion 8 times, accenting the *down* movement.

- On the last repetition, *hold* your leg up for 4 counts.

BACK OF THIGH
HAMSTRINGS

Step One:
WEIGHT PLACEMENT

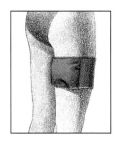

Place the weighted pouch of the Focus Weight cuff on the back of your right thigh midway between the knee and the hip. Secure it snugly so that it won't slip while you exercise.

ALIGNMENT: On all fours, when working with one leg extended to the rear, the hips should remain square and parallel to the floor and the back should be straight, not swayed. The knees should be separated and positioned directly under the hips. The hands should be placed directly under the shoulders. The head should align with the spine.

Step Two:
MOVEMENT

A. Kneel in an all-fours position, placing your hands directly under your shoulders. Extend your right leg out behind you with your toe pointed.

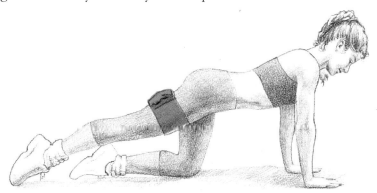

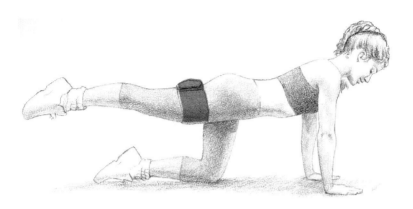

B. Keeping your hips and shoulders parallel to the floor and without bending your right knee, lift your right leg level with your hip. Pause.

Then lower your right leg almost to the floor.

Step Three:
REPETITIONS

> **TIP:** Avoid lifting your leg above hip height, as this can stress your lower back. Contract your buttocks with each lift.

- Repeat the full range of motion 8 times, accenting the *up* movement of your leg.

- Lift your right leg level with your hip. Maintaining this height and with a small range of motion, *pulse* your leg up and down 8 times.

- As you become stronger, increase the pulses to a maximum of 54.

- Lower and lift your leg 8 times in the full range of motion, accenting the *down* movement.

- *Hold* your leg up for 4 counts.

INNER THIGH
ADDUCTORS

Step One:
FOCUS WEIGHT PLACEMENT

Place the weighted pouch of the Focus Weight cuff on the inside of your right thigh midway between the knee and the hip. Secure it snugly so that it won't slip while you exercise.

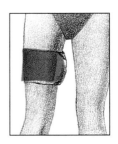

ALIGNMENT: Keep your abdominals contracted in order to prevent the back from swaying and to limit torso movement.

Step Two:
MOVEMENT

A. Kneel in an all-fours position, placing your hands directly under your shoulders. Hold your right leg straight out behind you at hip level. Bend your right leg to a 90° angle, keeping your thigh parallel to the ground.

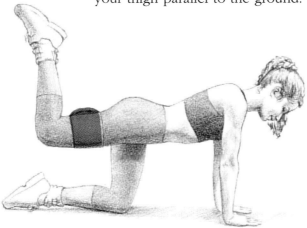

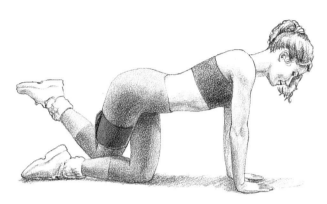

B. Drop and cross your right knee over your left calf. Pause. Then return your right knee to the starting position.

Step Three:
REPETITIONS

> **TIP:** Do not let your supporting side relax or slouch, especially when your working leg crosses over your supportive leg.

- Repeat the full range of motion 8 times, accenting the *crossing* motion of your leg.

- Cross your right knee over your left calf. Maintaining this position and with a small range of motion, *pulse* your leg up and across 8 times.

- As you become stronger, increase the pulses to a maximum of 54.

- Keeping your right leg bent at a 90° angle, lift it to hip level. Pause. Then drop your right knee across the left calf. Repeat the full range of motion 8 times, accenting the *up* movement.

- On the last repetition, *hold* your leg up for 4 counts.

Now that you have finished your right-leg workout, move the weight to your left leg and repeat the exercises. To cool down when you have completed the exercises with both legs, perform the stretching exercises described on pages 26–27.

WORKOUT #3: STANDING EXERCISES

This workout is done in a standing position with the use of a chair. The back of the chair should be at waist level. Keep your posture upright and your abdominals contracted. Don't lean on the chair: use it only to help you maintain balance.

Do all the exercises with your right leg first. Then switch legs and perform all the exercises with your left leg.

Before you begin, make sure you have had a proper warm-up/stretch and have completed the aerobic portion of your workout (if it's an aerobic day).

SCHEDULE AND ROUTINE

Warm-up/stretch	3–5 minutes
Aerobic activity	20–30 minutes, 3 times a week
Body sculpt	20 minutes daily
Repetitions	8–56 for each exercise
Cool-down/stretch	3–5 minutes

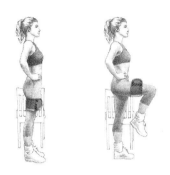

FRONT OF THIGH (Quadriceps)

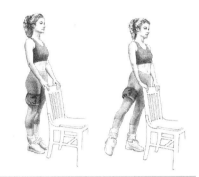

OUTER THIGH (Abductors)

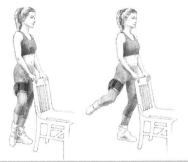

SADDLEBAG (Gluteus Medius)

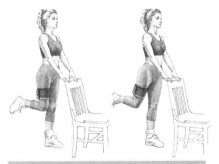

BACK OF THIGH (Hamstrings)

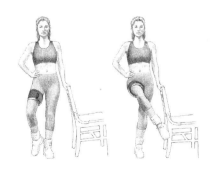

INNER THIGH (Adductors)

FRONT OF THIGH
QUADRICEPS

Step One:
FOCUS WEIGHT PLACEMENT

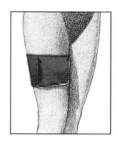

Place the weighted pouch of the Focus Weight cuff on the front part of your right thigh mid-way between the knee and the hip. Secure it snugly so that it won't slip while you exercise.

ALIGNMENT: In a standing position, keep your knees and toes facing forward. your hips should be slightly tucked under, the abdominals contracted, and your rib cage lifted. Shoulders should remain down and relaxed.

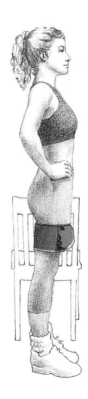

Step Two:
MOVEMENT

A. Standing with your left side to the chair, place your left hand on the chairback.

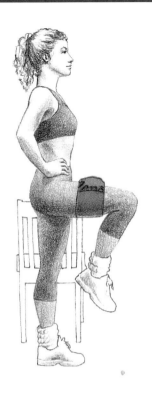

B. Lift your right knee level with your hip without altering your upper body position. Pause.

Then lower your right foot to the floor.

Step Three:
REPETITIONS

- Repeat the full range of motion 8 times, accenting the *up* movement of your leg.

- Lift your right knee to hip level. Maintaining this height and with a small range of motion, *pulse* your leg up and down 8 times.

- As you become stronger, increase the pulses to a maximum of 54.

> **TIP:** Don't lift your leg so high that your pelvis shifts out of alignment. In order to prevent strain to the hip flexors, never lift your working leg higher than your hip.

- Lower your right foot to the floor. Pause. Then lift your right knee level with your hip without altering your upper body position. Repeat the full range of motion 8 times, accenting the *down* movement.

- On the last repetition, *hold* your leg up for 4 counts.

OUTER THIGH
ABDUCTORS

Step One:
FOCUS WEIGHT PLACEMENT

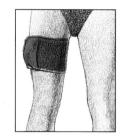

Place the weighted pouch of the Focus Weight cuff on the outside of your right thigh midway between the knee and the hip. Secure it snugly so that it won't slip while you exercise.

ALIGNMENT: In a standing position, keep your knees and toes facing forward. Your hips should be slightly tucked under, the abdominals contracted, and your rib cage lifted. Shoulders should remain down and relaxed.

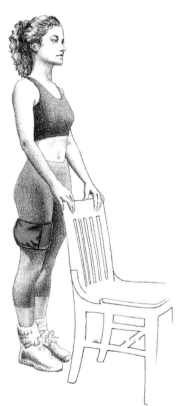

Step Two:
MOVEMENT

A: Standing behind the chair, place both hands on its back.

B: Keeping your feet parallel and your standing leg slightly bent, open your right leg as wide as you can without altering the alignment of your hips. Pause.

Then lower your leg to the starting position.

Step Three:

REPETITIONS

- Repeat the full range of motion 8 times, accenting the *outward* movement of your leg.

- Open your right leg out to the hip. Maintaining this height and with a small range of motion, *pulse* your leg out and in 8 times.

- As you become stronger, increase the pulses to a maximum of 54.

- Close and open your leg 8 times in the full range of motion, accenting the *inward* movement.

- On the last repetition, *hold* your leg out to the side for 4 counts.

> **TIP:** Your hips should remain square as you lift your working leg directly to the side while your knee faces forward. Your weight should be balanced evenly between your supporting leg and your working leg. Do not lean to the side to compensate for lack of strength or to achieve greater height.

SADDLEBAG

GLUTEUS MEDIUS

Step One:

FOCUS WEIGHT PLACEMENT

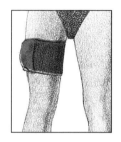

Place the weighted pouch of the Focus Weight cuff on the outside of your right thigh midway between the knee and the hip. Secure it snugly so that it won't slip while you exercise.

ALIGNMENT: Hold your torso still and erect while performing these exercises. Be sure to keep your shoulders and hips parallel to the back of the chair.

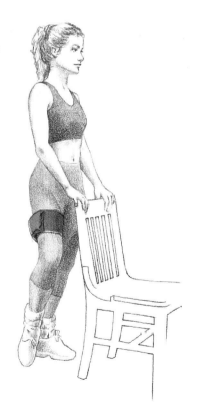

Step Two:

MOVEMENT

A. Standing behind the chair, place both hands on its back. Turn out your right leg from the hip, leaving your right knee slightly bent.

B. Keeping your hips square to the back of the chair, raise your right leg back in a diagonal movement. Pause.

Then lower your leg to the starting position.

Step Three:
REPETITIONS

- Repeat the full range of motion 8 times, accenting the *up* movement of your leg.

- Open your right leg back on the diagonal as far as you can without changing the alignment of the hips. Maintaining this height and with a small range of motion, *pulse* your leg back and forth 8 times.

> **TIP:** Even though your working leg is turned out, your hips should remain parallel to the back of the chair as you move your leg out and in on the diagonal. This will create the proper resistance.

- As you become stronger, increase the pulses to a maximum of 54.

- Leaving your right leg turned out from the hip, drop and lift your leg 8 times in the full range of motion, accenting the *down* movement.

- On the last repetition, *hold* your leg out for 4 counts.

BACK OF THIGH
HAMSTRINGS

Step One:
FOCUS WEIGHT PLACEMENT

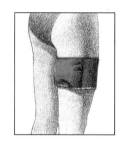

Place the weighted pouch of the Focus Weight cuff on the back of your right thigh midway between the knee and the hip. Secure it snugly so that it won't slip while you exercise.

ALIGNMENT: Do not lean forward into the chair but hold your body upright. Lift your leg straight back in the same line as the hip, keeping the knee facing forward so that the hamstring and buttock do the work.

Step Two:
MOVEMENT

A. Standing behind the chair, place both hands on its back.

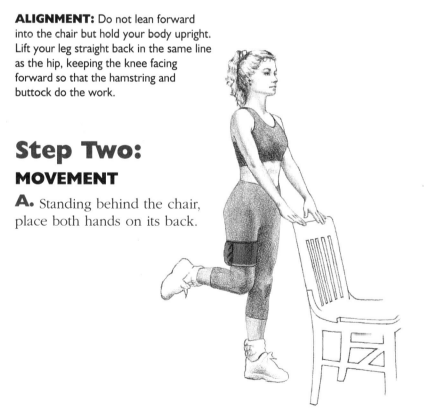

B. With your left foot facing the back of the chair, bend your right knee at a 90° angle. Push your bent right leg as far back as you can without altering the alignment of your hips. Pause.

Then return your leg to the starting position.

Step Three:
REPETITIONS

- Repeat the full range of motion 8 times, accenting the *backward* movement of your leg.

- Leave your right knee bent at a 90° angle and push your right leg back under the right buttock. Maintaining this height and with a small range of motion, *pulse* your leg back and forth 8 times.

- As you become stronger, increase the pulses to a maximum of 54.

- Leaving your right leg bent at a 90° angle, return your right knee to your left knee. Pause. Then push your right leg back under the right buttock. Repeat the full range of motion 8 times, accenting the *forward* movement.

- On the last repetition, *hold* your leg back for 4 counts.

TIP: In this position the range of motion is very limited. Do not push your working leg back beyond your buttock in order to prevent your back from hyperextending.

INNER THIGH
ADDUCTORS

Step One:
FOCUS WEIGHT PLACEMENT

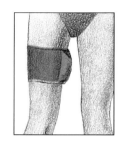

Place the weighted pouch of the Focus Weight cuff on the inside of your right thigh midway between the knee and the hip. Secure it snugly so that it won't slip while you exercise.

ALIGNMENT: Use the chair only for balance. Keep your body facing forward with your shoulders and hips aligned. Abdominals should be contracted.

Step Two:
MOVEMENT

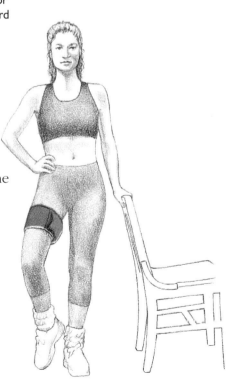

A. Stand with the back of the chair to your left. Place your left hand on the chairback. Lift your right leg slightly off the floor.

B. Keeping your hips facing forward, lift your right leg across your left leg in a diagonal motion. Pause.

Then lower your leg to the starting position.

Step Three:
REPETITIONS

• Repeat the full range of motion 8 times, accenting the *cross* movement of your leg.

• Lift your right leg up and across your left leg in a diagonal motion. Maintaining this height and with a small range of motion, *pulse* your leg up and across 8 times.

• As you become stronger, increase the pulse segment of the routine by 8 repetitions to a maximum of 54.

• Lower and lift your leg 8 times in the full range of motion, accenting the *down* movement.

• *Hold* your leg up and across for 4 counts.

TIP: Do not turn your hip or knee in as it crosses your body. This will allow one inner thigh to work against the other.

Now that you have finished your right-leg workout, move the weight to your left leg and repeat the exercises. To cool down when you have completed the exercises with both legs, perform the stretching exercises described on pages 26–27.

TEN TRAINING TIPS

I. Always check with your physician before beginning any exercise program.

2. Warm-up and stretch before you begin the sculpting program

3. If you are a beginner, perform 8-16 repetitions with each leg for each exercise. If you are a *moderate-level exerciser,* perform 16-32 repetitions with each leg for each exercise. If you are an *advanced exerciser,* perform 32-56 repetitions with each leg for each exercise.

4. Breathe evenly, exhaling as you lift and inhaling as you lower.

5. Work smoothly through the full range of motion described in each exercise. This will increase muscle strength

and maintain joint mobility.

6. Work at a steady, controlled pace. Be sure you use the muscle to do the work—be sure not to swing your legs or use momentum to do the lifts. Give yourself enough time to complete each lift fully.

7. Rest for 1-2 minutes between exercises.

8. For the quickest results, do the exercises *daily.*

9. Always cool down and stretch after every workout. It's important to lengthen the muscles to increase flexibility and alleviate muscle soreness.

10. If you do experience soreness, a warm bath may be soothing.

CHAPTER
4

NO BREAD,
NO BUBBLES

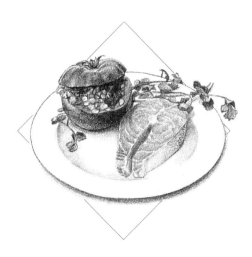

❏ NO BREAD, NO BUBBLES ... IT WORKED FOR ME

66 o Bread, no Bubbles" is the name I gave the eating plan that has proved effective for me and for many of my clients who wanted to reduce and reshape their thighs. "No Bread, no Bubbles" is a simple, commonsense method of planning your daily menus.

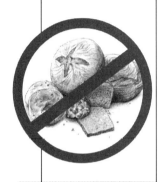

Before I go into the details, I want to tell you how I found the key to keeping my own body in the kind of shape that my profession as a fitness instructor requires. I have always had a healthy appetite and been a hearty eater. In my twenties I could eat anything I wanted, and what I wanted were pancakes or waffles for breakfast, two sandwiches for lunch, pasta or pizza for dinner. When I turned thirty, I found that my weight was going up and the sleek shape my career demanded was disappearing. Realizing that I would soon be out of a job if I didn't stop gaining, I knew I would have to make some changes in my eating habits.

> **Beware! Breads and pastas are foods that convert easily to sugar and then to body fat.**

When I took a careful look at my daily menus, I saw that breadlike starchy foods made up the preponderance of my diet. I was eating bagels, muffins, sandwiches, pasta, and pizza every day—three, four, or five times a day! The logical place to start making changes seemed to be in the area where was overindulging, so I wondered what would happen if I replaced breadlike starches with other foods.

> **A SENSIBLE CAUTION:** With this as with other eating plans, be sure to check with your doctor first.

I began to experiment with eggs, cheese, fruit, and/or yogurt for breakfast. I substituted salads—Greek salad, Caesar salad, chicken or tuna salad—for my lunchtime sandwiches, and at dinner I ate chicken, fish, beef, or turkey with green vegetables and salad instead of my usual pasta.

Within three days, I noticed that the bloating in my stomach had diminished, and within a week, I began to see changes in my thighs and hips. Excited and encouraged, I continued my new eating regime and soon regained the slim silhouette required by my work.

For me, I had found the key to weight control.

❏ SHARING THE KEY

My clients noticed the difference in the way I looked and asked me what kind of diet I was on. I told them that all I had done was to modify my menus by substituting other foods for starchy carbohydrates. Impressed by the changes they saw in me, my clients began to adopt breadless meals, too, and soon noticed a gratifying change in the feeling and appearance of their lower bodies.

What worked for me worked for other women, too!

❏ WHY IT WORKS: A SHORT LESSON IN NUTRITION

Curious to find out why my discovery worked, I spoke to several professionals in the field of nutrition. They explained the basic facts of carbohydrates (carbos), how they work in the body, and why a high-carbo diet may actually *undermine* efforts to lose weight.

73

"I have dropped bread from my diet and have lost 8 pounds in two weeks! It's delightful to finally have an answer to why I'd gained weight and how I can lose it and keep it off! I am eternally grateful!"
—Susan S., 41

All carbohydrates are sugars, and they are divided into two types. Simple carbohydrates are made up of either single or double sugar molecules and are found in candy, fruit and fruit juices, processed foods, and many soft drinks. Complex carbohydrates contain a large number of sugar molecules linked together in long chains. Foods like bread, cereal, rice, pasta, peas, and beans belong in this second group.

Simple sugars are released rapidly into the body and elevate blood sugar levels. The body reacts to this sudden inflow of sugar by secreting insulin into the bloodstream, not only shuttling fat into fat cells for storage but also preventing stored fat from being converted into energy. Because of these two insulin-induced reactions, simple sugar carbos that aren't being used are easily converted into body fat and should be limited or avoided if you are trying to lose weight.

Although complex carbohydrates are more nutritious and may not taste as sweet as simple sugars, they can also trip up a weight-loss program. If consumed in more than modest quantities, they provide more calories than the body can burn and they upset the insulin-sugar balance. Any carbos not immediately used by the body are stored as glycogen. The body's glycogen capacity is very limited, and when glycogen levels are full, the body converts the excess carbos into fat. Excess carbos are the enemy for people wanting to lose weight.

I also learned that the higher a food's carbohydrate count, the more insulin enters the bloodstream and the hungrier you feel. Some nutritionists recommend eating only protein and fruit for breakfast because the chemical makeup of a muffin or a bagel can trigger carbo bingeing. My experience with my clients taught me that while they did not crave and overeat apples and beans, they did crave bread and breadlike carbos such as pasta, rice, muffins, and pretzels.

My research helped me understand why omitting or cutting down on bread and breadlike foods seemed to work magic for me and my clients. In addition, it seemed only logical to me that, because women are genetically programmed to carry weight on their hips and thighs, excess fat ends up exactly where we don't want it!

My discovery, it turned out, was based on scientific fact.

❏ THE BUBBLE THEORY

Even though limiting breadlike carbos worked wonders for me and for many of my clients, I noticed that some women were not trimming down quite so quickly. I wondered why and asked them if they might be overindulging in something else. I soon discovered that many of them were drinking sodas or diet sodas or other carbonated beverages—sometimes as many as eight per day.

Employing my usual logical approach, I suggested that they substitute plain water or freshly brewed iced tea instead. In every single case they noticed an almost immediate end to the chronic bloating that had distressed them, and they, too, began to make rapid progress in slimming their problem areas!

The "no bubbles" part of my theory may be breaking new ground, but the fact is that limiting the intake of carbonated beverages has worked for many of my clients. Little research has been done in this area, but I

> Eliminate that bloated feeling by avoiding carbonated drinks, soda, and sparkling water. All introduce gas into your body via bubbles.

have discovered a few facts that seem to lend scientific support to my approach. A study done at the Southeast Baptist Hospital in San Antonio, Texas, discovered that one can of soda contains up to 1,000 cubic centimeters of dissolved carbon dioxide. A thousand cubic centimeters equals a liter. Quick math shows that drinking three or four sodas a day puts 3 or 4 liters of carbon dioxide into the stomach. No wonder my clients looked swollen and felt bloated!

In addition, carbonated drinks containing sugar trigger the insulin-producing/fat-storing response and the appetite-stimulating effects of carbos. There is also evidence that the artificial sweeteners used in diet sodas trick the body into thinking that it has consumed sugar, thus evoking the same insulin-producing/fat-storing responses. If you drink a lot of soda, either regular or diet, and are having trouble controlling your weight, try replacing carbonated beverages with plain water or freshly brewed iced tea.

> Drink at least 8 glasses of water a day! The more you drink, the more the body will excrete. Drink too little and the body will retain all the fluid it can, thus causing a puffy appearance.

❏ R$_x$: WATER

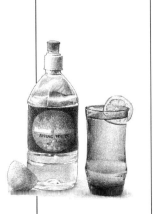

I recommend drinking at least eight 8-ounce glasses of plain water a day to help in the digestion of food and the metabolism of fat. Water gives you a feeling of fullness without the gas contributed by carbonated beverages, and, at the same time, it helps flush out bodily wastes, including by-products from the breakdown of fat. The nutritionists I consulted told me that if these by-products are not eliminated from the system, the body slows down the rate at which it burns fat.

Once you make a habit of drinking enough plain

water every day, you will notice that you feel better and look slimmer!

❏ A SIMPLE PLAN TO CONTROL YOUR WEIGHT

Based on my own experience and that of my clients, bread and bubbles are the double whammy every thigh-conscious woman should beware of! Try these two temporary modifications in your present menus: limit bread or breadlike carbos; and avoid beverages containing bubbles. The next few pages will get you started, giving you sample menus, and showing you how to reshape your body without being miserable or starving yourself.

❏ YOUR OWN FOOD AND DRINK DIARY

For one day, keep a food and drink diary. Write down everything you eat and drink: meals, snacks, nibbles, and liquids. Then, add up the number of bread or bread-like carbos and the number of diet sodas and carbon-ated beverages you consumed.

What follows is the before and after diary of one of my clients. An asterisk represents one carbo serving, a plus symbol, a carbonated drink. When I analyzed the before chart, I saw that Carol had had 17 carbos and 4 bubbly drinks that day. She was shocked to realize that she had been consuming some version (and usually more than one) of bread and/or bubbles all day long.

FOOD FACTS AND SNACKING STRATEGIES

1. Always eat three meals a day and, if you get hungry between meals, snack on anything that appeals to you from the list of suggested foods on page 80.

2. It's old advice, but so true: eat s-l-o-w-l-y so that your body has a chance to feel satisfied.

3. It is important not to feel deprived. Be sure to choose foods that you like in your new eating plan.

4. Many of the low-fat or no-fat snacks you may have been eating are dangerous to your thighs! Some of the biggest offenders my clients have mentioned are pretzels, popcorn, crackers, melba toast, "lite" chips, granola bars, dry cereal, and rice cakes all breadlike carbos.

5. Try to eat something every 4 hours. Don't let yourself get hungry, because your blood sugar will plummet and you will be tempted to stuff yourself.

I modified Carol's eating plan so that she could still have three full meals plus two snacks and one dessert a day. Her new "after" eating plan reduces her carbo intake by half and replaces all her breadlike carbos with with starchless choices. She was never hungry, she ate delicious and healthful foods, and she noticed the difference in her hips and thighs almost immediately.

If, after examining your own food and drink diary, you find that you have been consuming too much bread and too many bubbles, begin the program by eliminating most if not all of them from your diet and substituting other foods such as the ones on page 80 in their place. Changing your habits will be much easier than you think. When you decrease the amount of bread and

CAROL'S FOOD DIARY

BEFORE

BREAKFAST: *orange juice • bagel* • coffee*

MORNING SNACK: *4 rice cakes**** • an apple • diet soda+*

LUNCH: *• tuna sandwich** • potato chips* • pasta salad* • diet soda+*

AFTERNOON SNACK: *small bag of pretzels* • 3 lowfat oatmeal raisin cookies*** • diet soda+*

DINNER: *hamburger with bun** • french fries* • cole slaw • diet soda+ • carrot cake**

AFTER

BREAKFAST: *orange juice • lowfat yogurt with blueberries** • coffee*

MORNING SNACK: *peach* • skim-milk cappuccino*

LUNCH: *lentil soup* • Greek salad • fresh-brewed iced tea*

AFTERNOON SNACK: *sugar-free Jell-O • assorted raw nuts such as almonds or peanuts* • coffee or tea*

DINNER: *shrimp cocktail • chicken • spinach* • acorn squash* • raspberry sherbet*

(We've used * for number of servings of carbos and + for bubbles.)

carbonated drinks you consume, your cravings for them will be dramatically reduced! Within three or four days, a new, slimmer look and feeling will be your reward.

❏ BREAD REPLACEMENTS

Because you want to limit only bread and breadlike foods, you are free to choose from other food groups such as protein, dairy, fruits, and vegetables. Be warned, though, that fruit and fruit juice are simple sugars, and you should have no more than three per day. Try to choose low-fat dairy products, unsweetened desserts, and "lite," salad dressings. When you cook food, grill, broil, bake, or steam rather than fry.

I've already shown you one sample meal chart but, because it is important to vary your diet, here are some more suggestions to help you get started on your new eating plan.

Breakfast: boiled, scrambled, or poached eggs; Western omelet or egg-white omelet with cheese and/or vegetables; melon with cottage cheese; fruit with yogurt; fresh fruit salad; sugar-free protein breakfast shake (available in health food stores).

Lunch: soup (your choice); salad with protein (chicken, turkey, tofu, poached or smoked fish), Caesar salad; Greek salad; chili; baked potato with a low-fat or vegetable topping; hamburger (no bun); tuna, shrimp, or chicken salad platter; tomato stuffed with egg, tuna, shrimp, or chicken salad.

Dinner: fish or shellfish; turkey; lamb; veal; lean red meat; or chicken; your choice of vegetables from the chart on page 80 plus a salad; dessert such as sher-

> Don't skip meals! When you don't eat regularly, the body goes into a "starvation mode." Not knowing if or when it will be nourished again, it conserves energy and does not burn calories.

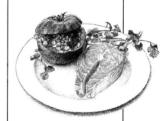

79

ARE THERE ANY CARBOS I CAN HAVE?

Although I am suggesting that you temporarily eliminate bread and breadlike foods from your meals, it is important to include in your diet carbohydrates such as those in fruits, legumes, and vegetables. You can and should eat some of the following every day:

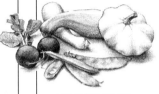

VEGETABLES

- *artichokes*
- *asparagus*
- *broccoli*
- *brussels sprouts*
- *cabbage*
- *carrots*
- *cauliflower*
- *celery*
- *collard greens*
- *corn*
- *cucumbers*
- *eggplant*
- *green peas*
- *leeks*
- *lettuce or other leafy greens*
- *onions*
- *potatoes (baked or steamed)*
- *red and green peppers*
- *spinach*
- *squash*
- *string beans*
- *tomatoes*
- *yams*
- *zucchini*

LEGUMES

- *black beans*
- *black-eyed peas*
- *kidney beans*
- *garbanzo beans*
- *lentils*
- *lima beans*
- *navy beans*
- *pinto beans*

FRUIT

- *apples*
- *bananas*
- *blackberries*
- *blueberries*
- *cantaloupe*
- *cherries*
- *grapefruit*
- *honeydew*
- *mangoes*
- *nectarines*
- *oranges*
- *papayas*
- *peaches*
- *pears*
- *pineapple*
- *plums*
- *raspberries*
- *strawberries*
- *tangerines*
- *watermelon*

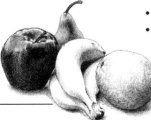

bet; Jell-O; frozen yogurt; yogurt-berry parfait; or frozen fruit on a stick.

Snacks: fresh fruit; yogurt; raw nuts and pumpkin or sunflower seeds; vegetables with low-fat dip; olives; pickles; cottage cheese (plain or flavored); cold cuts; cheese; flavored tea or coffee.

❏ A WORD ABOUT PORTIONS

As long as it isn't bread or bubbles, you can have it and then some. Because you have eliminated these two food categories from your diet, you may find that you are eating larger portions of other foods to help fill you up. Go ahead, and don't worry about it. Just use common sense and moderation as your guides.

For example, if the choice is between a large salad and a small one and you are hungry, go ahead and have the large one. In addition, the difference between two slices of chicken or turkey and three is insignificant. However, when it comes to snacks, salad dressings, and desserts that contain fat or sugar, proceed with caution. If the choice is between a large frozen yogurt and a small one, have the small one.

❏ BREAD-AND-BUBBLE BONUS

You may be wondering if you can ever have bread again. The answer is . . . *yes!*

> Sit down when you eat—even your snacks. Eating on the run lends itself to bread-like snacks like bagels, crackers, pretzels, popcorn and so on.

> Be sure to eat plenty of vegetables and beans. They are a great source of fiber and minerals.

REALITY CHECK
Although I am suggesting that you temporarily eliminate bread and breadlike foods from your meals, it is important to include in your diet carbohydrates such as those in fruits, legumes, and vegetables. You can and should eat some of them every day.

Once you have attained the shape you want, add one breadlike carbo or carbonated beverage a week to your diet. See whether or not you maintain your new shape. If you do, add a second breadlike carbo or carbonated beverage to your weekly menus and see what happens. If you still maintain your new shape, add a third, and so on. When you find that your thighs are beginning to balloon again, stop!

Somewhere between completely avoiding bread and bubbles and your previous eating habits lies a safe quantity for your personal maintenance program.

When you have determined how much bread and/or bubbles you can consume, keep a mental list and stay within your limits. Replace one choice with another whenever necessary. For example, if you go to a birthday party and have a piece of cake, substitute it for one of your other bread or breadlike foods that week.

❏ TEMPTATIONS AND INDULGENCES

My No-Bread, No-Bubbles food strategy is a guideline, not a rigid commandment of do's and don'ts. There are situations in life—a party, a fabulous restaurant, a vacation—when we give in to temptation. I have and I will! You have and you will!

Do your best to keep your indulgences within your own personal carbo limits, but when you do fall off the wagon, there is no point in feeling guilty or in berating yourself. Just go back to the No-Bread, No-Bubbles plan or your own personal maintenance program as soon as you can.

❏ LOOK NO FURTHER

My Thighs to Die For Program will work for you, and, when it does, you, too, will have found the key to controlling your shape.

Just as it is crucial to be able to see the changes in your body when they happen, it is important to stop searching for other answers once you discover what works for you. The next fad diet, pill, or gimmick is not going to be any better than others have been in the past. You now have the key to weight and shape control, and, if you find that your lower body is getting heavy again, all you have to do is return to the Thighs to Die For Program. You already know it works!